Don Green
2280 Ardmore Cove
Memphis, TN. 38127
U.S.A   357-7444

DID YOU KNOW . . .

that garlic can help prevent and correct the following conditions:

- HIGH BLOOD PRESSURE
- HEART DISEASE
- DIABETES
- ARTHRITIS
- CANCER
- EMPHYSEMA
- DIGESTIVE DISORDERS
- INTESTINAL WORMS
- INSOMNIA
- COLDS
- ALLERGIES
- ASTHMA
- and many others

W9-BUI-208

In this book, Dr. Paavo Airola, internationally recognized nutritionist and leading exponent of biological medicine, reports on reputable scientific research and clinical studies which demonstrate the remarkable preventive and healing properties of garlic.

The Miracle of

Garlic

**Worldwide scientific studies reveal the
amazing nutritional and medicinal properties
of a common, but much neglected,
"wonder food"**

by PAAVO AIROLA, N.D., Ph.D.

HEALTH PLUS, PUBLISHERS
P.O. Box 22001, Phoenix, Arizona 85028

First printing, January, 1978
Second printing, March, 1978
Third printing, July, 1978
Fourth printing, December, 1978
Fifth printing, July, 1979
Sixth printing, January, 1980
Seventh printing, June, 1980
Eighth printing, April, 1981

IMPORTANT NOTES:

This book does not intend to diagnose or prescribe—the information in it is presented for educational purposes only and is best used in cooperation with your doctor. In the event the reader uses the information to solve his own health problems, he is prescribing for himself, which is his constitutional right, but the author and the publisher assume no responsibility.

Also, I wish to stress the fact that I do not sell, nor have any financial or economic interest in foods or supplements mentioned or recommended in this publication. The sole reason for writing this book is to help the readers, the members of the healing professions, the researchers, and the serious students of nutrition and natural healing by giving them vital information about garlic and its nutritional and medicinal properties which I have uncovered through years of study and research.

The Author

Printed in the U.S.A.

TABLE OF CONTENTS:

INTRODUCTION 7
GARLIC: POISON OR MIRACLE FOOD 11
    Why Nutrition Confusion 11
    Outdated Information 12
    The Price of Freedom 13
EMPIRICAL EVIDENCE 14
MODERN RESEARCH ON GARLIC 16
    High Blood Pressure 16
    Atherosclerosis and Heart Disease 17
    Anemia 18
    Rheumatic Diseases 18
    Diabetes 19
    Hypoglycemia 19
ANTIBIOTIC PROPERTY OF GARLIC 20
ANTIBACTERIAL AND ANTIFUNGAL PROPERTIES OF GARLIC 20
ANTICANCER PROPERTY OF GARLIC 21
    Germanium and Cancer 21
GARLIC: THE MIRACLE HEALER 22
OTHER CLINICAL USES OF GARLIC 23
• Eye burns • Lip and mouth diseases • Coagulation disorders • Upset stomach • Hyperemia • Grippe • Sciatica • Chronic colitis • Gastritis • Whooping cough • Beriberi • Pimples • Emphysema • Athletes' foot • Worms • Constipation • Intestinal disorders • Colds

PESTICIDAL PROPERTIES OF GARLIC 27
ANIMAL DISEASES AND GARLIC ....
ANTIOXIDANT PROPERTY OF GARLIC 28
GARLIC: POWERFUL DETOXIFIER 29

HEAVY METAL POISONING AND GARLIC 30
HOW AND WHY GARLIC WORKS 32
THE CHEMICAL AND NUTRITIONAL COMPOSITION OF GARLIC 34
DELICIOUS GOURMET FOOD 35
GARLIC AND COMMON SENSE 36
    "If he kissed you once, will he kiss you again?" 36
    Great News From Japan 37
QUESTIONS AND ANSWERS 39
CONCLUSION 43
REFERENCES 44

INTRODUCTION

Nutritionally speaking, we are living in the most exciting era of man's history—a time of great *nutrition awareness*. For centuries, orthodox medicine, blinded by the erroneous and outdated Pasteurian concept of the bacterial origin of disease, has kept us in darkness regarding the role that our life style, and specifically our nutrition, plays in our health and our disease. The prevailing conventional medical concept of disease is that bacteria or germs are vicious invaders that attack healthy organisms in their way and cause various diseases—each disease depending on the kind of invading bacteria.

Throughout medical history, the philosophies and concepts of disease and the approved methods of healing have changed with almost every generation. At one time, doctors believed that disease was caused by demons. Later generations of doctors used blood letting as a cure-all, since "bad blood" was considered to be the cause of all disease. Although accepted philosophies of disease have varied with nearly every generation, somehow orthodox medicine has never seriously considered Hippocrates' philosophy of health and disease: that most ills are of man's own making and are the result of his violation of the elementary rules of health. So, when Pasteur came up with the bacteria theory, it was met with immediate acceptance. The germ theory removed health maintenance and disease prevention from the domain of man himself and put it in the doctor's hands. The idea that they are the only ones able to defend mankind from vicious germs appealed to doctors.

The complete fiasco of today's orthodox medicine and its germ concept of disease is evidenced by the fact that in spite of more doctors, more and better equipped hospitals, more germ-killing drugs, and more money spent on health care (actually "disease care") than at any time in man's history, *we have more disease than ever before.* We are witnessing a catastrophic increase in all the chronic degenerative conditions, including heart disease, arthritis, diabetes, and cancer. In fact, according to official statistics published by the medical establishment, almost half of all Americans are chronically ill! Heart disease alone kills over one million Americans each year

While orthodox drug- and knife-oriented doctors are unable to cope with the increased amount of disease, people are beginning to lose faith in them. They are turning to unorthodox healers—doctors of biological medicine, doctors who restore health by correcting man's eating and living habits, not by combatting germs with toxic drugs. These "new breed of doctors" are now known as practicing preventive, orthomolecular, metabolic, nutritional, botanical (herbal), manipulative, holistic, or biological medicine. These doctors recognize that while the basic causes of disease are to be found in man's own health-destroying eating and living habits, likewise the cure for all disease is inherent in the body's own healing power. The doctor of biological medicine does not cure disease. He helps a sick body cure itself by strengthening the patient's resistance and supporting the body's own healing activity with various biological means, such as improved diet, herbs, vitamins, fasting, rest, relaxation, exercise, positive health-oriented mental attitude, etc. Biological Medicine puts the blame for man's ills on man's own eating and living habits and his disregard for the elementary laws of good health. Likewise, the responsibility for the prevention and correction of disease is placed upon man himself, on his own positive and constructive health-building and disease-preventive efforts. A disease-ridden mankind can finally rejoice and benefit from the fact that the Dark Age of Pasteurian germ-concept medicine, with its deadly chemical drugs, serums, X-rays, vaccines, burning and cutting, is finally well on its way to being replaced by a new, holistic approach to healing—the healing science of the New Age, *Biological Medicine.*

Nutrition: Foundation for Optimum Health

More and more people, disenchanted with the conventional doctors' inability to cope with the catastrophic increase in degenerative, crippling and killing diseases, are taking health into their own hands or turning to the unconventional healers. They are becoming aware that nutrition, so long ignored and/or ridiculed by their family physician, is an important factor in their well-being. They are discovering that "they are what they eat," that what they eat is definitely related to the way they feel—to their level of vitality, energy, and resistance to disease. This sudden and massive American "nutrition awareness" is, perhaps, the most unique and far-reaching phenomenon in the concluding decades of the twentieth century, overshadowing in importance most other events that make the headlines. Once the fact that optimum nutrition *is* one of the most important factors in prevention of disease will be recognized by most Americans, the catastrophic deterioration of our health will finally be halted, and we can begin to look forward to long and happy disease-free lives.

Those who have been health- and nutrition-oriented for some time are aware that the concept of *optimum nutrition* in this age of universal pollution, toxic environment, and steadily deteriorating quality of foods means more than just eating an "adequate diet" composed of "four basic food groups." Supplementing any diet with vitamins, minerals, and special food supplements is now recognized as a must to assure optimum nutrition and an adequate protection against disease and against the toxic chemicals in our polluted food, water, air, and environment. Health seekers have discovered that certain natural foods, often referred to as "wonder foods" or "super foods," are excellent food supplements which contain concentrated nutrition, and supply in abundnace certain nutrients and other factors that are often missing in a regular diet. Thus, such foods as wheat germ, brewers yeast, yogurt, dessicated liver, cod liver oil, garlic, seaweed (kelp), bone meal, and bran have become "regular" additions to the optimum diet.

This book takes a close look at one of these "wonder foods" —garlic. In my life-long study of nutrition, I have become more and more aware of the miraculous health-building, disease-preventing, and healing properties contained in this well-known aromatic vegetable, which is so ignored in American nutrition. I hope that after reading this small book you will become, as I am, an enthusiastic connoisseur and epicure of garlic, and will incorporate it into your daily diet, especially so in view of the fact that now the factor that has prevented most of us from eating garlic on a regular basis—its strong odor—has been removed from some of the available garlic supplements, which will enable everyone to eat this miracle food without social limitations.

Hippocrates, the "Father of Medicine," perhaps the greatest healer that ever lived, wrote 2500 years ago:

> "Let your food be your medicine—
> let your medicine be your food."

Garlic, more than any other food, fits into Hippocrates' description of an ideal food: that which is both a super-nutritious food and a miracle medicine!

You will find that the following discourse is not just an enthusiastic endorsement of garlic by a garlic lover, but a fully-documented study based on an impressive amount of material from reliable university and clinical studies and research from several continents. It could be, therefore, truthfully said that the nutritional and therapeutic value of garlic is not only proven by the empirical evidence during thousands of years of universal use, both as food and a medicine, but also by irrefutable worldwide scientific research.

Paavo Airola, Ph.D.

GARLIC: POISON OR MIRACLE FOOD?

From the readers of "Nutrition Forum," my monthly column in **New Realities** Magazine, and from the readers of my books, I receive hundreds of questions every week. Some of them deal with personal health problems, some with general or specific questions in the field of nutrition. I receive many questions regarding the value of garlic. It seems that some writers and nutrition "experts" are trying to discredit one of mankind's most well-known and cherished foods. Here is one of the letters I recently received:

> Dear Dr. Airola:
>
> In your books, you highly recommend garlic. In fact, in *ARE YOU CONFUSED?*, you refer to garlic as "the king of the vegetable kingdom" and mention many studies and clinical tests that demonstrate garlic's almost miraculous healing and health-building properties. Yet, I just read a book by another famous writer who says that garlic is poison and should never be eaten in any form. Who is right? Why such disagreement between two experts, both of whom I consider to be leaders in the fields of nutrition and holistic medicine? Please, help me to find out the truth. Give me the facts!
>
> Ms. P. F., Hollywood, CA.

Why Nutrition Confusion

You don't have to read far into American so-called health literature to discover that there is a great diversity of opinion on many pertinent questions related to nutrition and health. There are many reasons for this. The almighty dollar—greedy commercialism—is, perhaps, the prime reason. Many experts are involved in manufacturing and selling the products and services which they so highly recommend. It is difficult to be totally objective when you have an axe to grind. Also, medicine and nutrition are not exact sciences. Every vitamin or food brings a different reaction in each individual, and, therefore, it is often difficult to draw a generalized conclusion. Scholastic dogmatism in the area of human nutrition, the scientifically rigid adherence to a principle or tenet, without taking the varied and changeable human element into consideration, can only result in pseudo-science and confusion.

Moreover, not only is the study material human and varied, but nutritionists and health writers are human, too. They may be very subjective in their judgement. Many of their conclusions and beliefs may be colored by their own likes and dislikes. For example, the son of one of the most knowledgeable and prolific health writers and respected nutritionists, now deceased, wrote that his father's strong pro-meat, high-protein stand was motivated by his own personal liking for the taste of meat!

There is also a deplorable lack of dependable research on nutrition in our country. Almost all nutrition research, whether in private research centers or universities, is done and/or financed by the giant commercial food industries involved. And, "he who pays the piper calls the tune." Just a hypothetical example: it would be naive to expect that research on the nutritional value of sugar, financed by the sugar industry, would turn up revealing facts that refined sugar is a mass killer—which, in fact, it is.

Outdated Information

Another point to consider is that although nutrition is as old as mankind, the *science of nutrition* is a relatively new field of research. It has been said that we have learned more about nutrition in the last 20 years than in the preceding 2000 years.

For example, the idea that garlic and onions are poisonous foods originated with the writings of some natural hygienists more than a half a century ago, then was repeated by some of their followers in more recent times. Their conclusions were based on outdated, obsolete beliefs and speculations rather than on scientific data. Since then, Russian, Finnish, Indian, Japanese, and American research has shown that garlic and onions are miracle health-promoting and disease-preventing foods, as I will show later in this book.

The Price of Freedom

For several decades now, Americans have been obsessed with self-criticism and fault-finding, seemingly oblivious to the fact that in spite of our imperfections—political corruption, high crime rate, inflation, etc.—the United States is still, and by far, the best, the safest, and the freest country in the world. Not only do we have the highest living standard in the world, but we have more personal freedoms and basic human rights than any nation on earth. But, even freedom has its price. Nutrition confusion is just one of the prices we must pay for living in a free country, where there is a free press and guaranteed freedom of expression—i.e., where anyone can write books and pose as an expert. One of our most knowledgeable nutritionists, Dr. Carlton Fredericks, hit the nail on the head when he said, "everyone who eats thinks he is an authority on nutrition." Consequently, we have a growing number of book-writing "authorities," who present their dramatically opposing and contradictory views on virtually any given subject, leaving their readers and followers wallowing in total confusion and bewilderment. I don't know how we could remedy this situation without infringement on our highly cherished freedom of expression and freedom of the press. I guess the reader just has to make his own choice of experts and nutritional gurus, and follow the ideas and advice that make the *most sense to him or her.*

But, in the reader's question cited earlier, I was asked for facts; facts that substantiate my enthusiastic endorsement of garlic as a miraculous healing and health-building food. So, let's hear the facts.

EMPIRICAL EVIDENCE

Garlic has been used for thousands of years both as food and as medicine. Most people around the world, especially those known for their excellent health, absence of disease, and long life, have used, and are now using, garlic extensively in their daily diets. I have studied the diets of Russians and Bulgarians, where onions and garlic are consumed in astronomical quantities. Not a single case of garlic poisoning has ever been known among them. On the contrary, healthy Russian centenarians often have told me that the large amount of garlic and onions in their diets was one of the main causes of their exceptional health and long life.

According to the Old Testament, one of the chief complaints of the children of Israel on one of their many long journeys was that they had no garlic with them. Ancient Egyptian records show that the pyramid builders had raw garlic as part of their food ration; when hard-working pyramid builders threatened to leave the pyramids unfinished, the Pharaoh stimulated their incentive to continue with increased rations of garlic.[1] The Pharaoh spent the equivalent of nearly two million dollars buying garlic to feed the workers who built the great Cheops pyramid. The Vikings and the Phoenicians, warriors and adventurers, packed garlic in their sea chests when they started on their lengthy sea voyages.

Garlic has also been attributed with miraculous healing powers, and used throughout medical history in the treatment of many kinds of disease. Ancient records show that garlic was used as medicine as early as 3000 B.C. by Babylonians, Chinese, Greeks, Romans, Egyptians, and Vikings. Most great physicians of old—Pliny, Dioscorides, Hippocrates, and Galen, to name a few—as well as some more contemporary medical greats such as Are Waerland, Werner Zabel, Ragnar Berg, Albert Schweitzer, Bircher-Benner, and many others, used garlic to cure everything from intestinal infections and digestive disorders to high blood pressure, senility, and impotence.[2]

Pliny, ancient Roman naturalist and physician, listed 61 diseases that could be effectively treated with garlic. He said, "Garlic has such powerful properties that the very smell of it drives away serpents and scorpions." Pliny claimed that garlic has curative power in all respiratory and tubercular ailments.

According to the Talmud, the eating of garlic was recommended for many reasons: "it satiates hunger, it brightens up the face, it improves circulation and keeps the body warm," and it kills the parasites. The Romans gave garlic to their hard laborers to "impart strength" and to their soldiers to "incite courage." The Irish, Danish, and Russians used garlic for centuries as a treatment for coughs and colds. In Ireland, chronic bronchitis was treated with garlic by old-time physicians. Dr. W. T. Fernie, in an old medical book, *Meals Medicinal,* tells of garlic being effectively used to treat many diseases, including whooping cough and tuberculosis. He tells of a doctor who gave garlic to all his gall bladder patients. He also said that "a garlic clove, when introduced into the bowel, will destroy thread worms, and, if eaten, will abolish round worms."

During World War I, the British Army used garlic to control infections in wounds. The raw garlic juice was diluted with water and applied directly to the wounds with excellent results.[3] The same method was practiced by Russian army doctors during World War II. Garlic and onions were given internally to increase resistance against infections, as well as used externally to speed the healing of wounds.

MODERN RESEARCH ON GARLIC

When I began the research for this book, I found to my amazement that there has been a tremendous amount of scientific garlic research done in various parts of the world. After reading the following research reports, you will be convinced, as I was, that they clearly confirm the ancient beliefs, "old wives' tales," and enthusiastic claims by the folk medicine healers regarding the therapeutic and preventive properties of garlic.

High Blood Pressure

One of the conditions in which garlic treatment brings the fastest and clearly measurable improvements is hypertension, or high blood pressure. In my own clinical practice, I have treated many patients with high blood pressure; in most cases the blood pressure was reduced 20–30 mm. in one week by taking large amounts of garlic or garlic preparations.

Dr. F. G. Piotrowski, of the University of Geneva, used garlic on patients with abnormally high blood pressure. The study revealed that garlic treatment brought "excellent results." Garlic, according to Dr. Piotrowski, has a dilating effect on blood vessels, and, thus, is effective in reducing blood pressure.[4] Dr. Piotrowski used garlic on about 100 patients. In 40% of the cases he obtained a drop of 20 mm. in blood pressure after about a week of garlic treatment. The subjective symptoms, such as dizziness, angina-like pain, headaches, and backaches, began to disappear 3–5 days after the start of the garlic treatment.

A study in India, conducted under the direction of Drs. Sainani, Desai, and More, showed that garlic and onions have a preventive effect on the development of arteriosclerosis and consequent high blood pressure and heart disease.[5]

From the experiments on both animals and humans, Drs. Debray and Loeper found that garlic tincture causes a decided drop in blood pressure in most cases of hypertension.[6]

The German pharmaceutical journal reported on recent animal and human studies by V. Petkov to determine clinical and pharmacological effects of garlic. In high blood pressure studies on cats, intravenous injections of 0.05 g./kg. of garlic extract (corresponding to 0.20 g. of garlic) lowered blood pressure 50 mm. In studies on dogs with experimentally induced hypertension, garlic reduced their systolic pressure "significantly." And in clinical human studies on 114 patients having hypertension and atherosclerosis, garlic caused a marked improvement in the systolic (8-33 mm.) and diastolic arterial tension (4-20 mm.).[7]

Atherosclerosis and Heart Disease

Pathologist Dr. R. C. Jain, of the University of Benghazi in Libya, demonstrated in experimental animal studies that garlic can prevent plaque formation in arteries and, thus, help prevent the development of atherosclerosis and heart disease.[8]

Drs. Arun Bordia and H. C. Bansal, Indian researchers, reported in the respected British medical journal, *Lancet,* on human studies designed to evaluate the effect of garlic oil on cholesterol and triglyceride levels in the blood. They fed one fourth pound of butter at one time to five healthy volunteers. This is enough to raise cholesterol and other fatty substances in the blood considerably. As expected, three hours after the volunteers had eaten the butter, their cholesterol levels had risen from an average of 221.4 to 237.4. Later, the same volunteers received the same amount of butter along with the juice of 50 grams of garlic. This time, the cholesterol level, instead of rising, went down from 228.7 to 212.7 in three hours.[1]

Two other researchers from the Department of Biochemistry at the University of Kerala, India, Dr. K. T. Augusti and P. T. Mathew, reported the results of their recent garlic studies on rats. They fed allicin (the active sulfur-containing compound in garlic that is changed into diallyldisulphide in the system) to normal rats for a period of 2 months. The result was that the garlic reduced the lipid levels in the serum and the liver "significantly."[9]

In human studies, it has been observed that a long-term daily administration of garlic juice to hypercholesterolaemic patients (dose: 0.5 ml./kg.), lowered the serum cholesterol levels considerably.[10]

The above-cited study by Augusti et al., showed that allicin (from garlic) seemed to have a marked effect on certain processes of synthesis or breakdown of lipids in the liver. On a long-term administration, it significantly reduced the lipid levels in the serum and liver of normal rats. This may explain the therapeutic value of garlic when it is used in the treatment of heart disease and atherosclerosis. Excessive lipids (fatty substances such as triglycerides and cholesterol) in the arteries are considered to be the major contributing cause of heart disease and heart attacks.[8]

Anemia

A controlled Australian study by Dr. K. Halwax showed that garlic extract (odorless liquid garlic extract, Kyolic) has a beneficial effect in the treatment of anemia. Studies show that the hemoglobin and red cell count were significantly higher in the group of 10 female patients with chronic anemia after 8 weeks of treatment, as compared to 10 patients with the same degree of anemia who were given placebos.[11]

Warning: Note that the above research was done with liquid garlic extract, not raw garlic. There is some evidence that *excessively* large amounts of *raw* garlic in the diet may contribute to the development of anemia. Therefore, anemic patients should take only garlic extracts or garlic in cooked form, not in raw form.

Rheumatic Diseases

In Japan, the Department of Surgery at Fukuyama Army Hospital of Self Defense Force, tested the same garlic extract (Kyolic) on patients with lumbago and arthritis. The extract showed "remarkable" effectiveness on 86% of the patients.[12] No undesirable side effects were observed.

It has been shown in animal studies that garlic exhibits some antiinflammatory activity, which accounts for its effectiveness in the treatment of arthritis.[13] Allisotin, prepared from garlic (200 mg./100 g./day), was found effective in study rats against an inflammatory arthritis condition induced by Formalin (formaldehyde).

Diabetes

It has been demonstrated in many animal and human studies that garlic is one of the few completely natural and harmless substances which are effective in the treatment of diabetes, or high blood sugar.

Three physicians from India, Drs. Jain, Vyas, and Mahatma, reported in *Lancet,* the British medical journal, that onion and garlic juice was given to rabbits which had first been made diabetic. The result was that their high blood sugar levels were brought down quickly.[14] Some doctors reported earlier experiments (1958) which showed that garlic and onions are effective in reducing blood sugar levels.[1]

Hypoglycemia

Hypoglycemia means *low* blood sugar—the opposite of diabetes, which is high blood sugar. However, garlic seems to affect hypoglycemia favorably also. It has been demonstrated that several of the common sulfur-containing compounds of garlic have special sugar metabolism regulating factors, which can help normalize both high and low blood sugar levels. Garlic is also an excellent detoxifier; it improves the general metabolism and has a stimulating effect on the liver, the nervous system, and the circulation. Garlic strengthens the body's defenses against allergens (foods one is allergic to); and hypoglycemics often suffer from allergies.[15,16]

ANTIBIOTIC PROPERTY OF GARLIC

Russian electrobiologist, Professor Gurwitch, discovered that garlic emits a peculiar type of ultra-violet radiation called mitogenetic radiations. These emissions, now referred to as Gurwitch rays, have the property of stimulating cell growth and activity and have a rejuvenative effect on all body functions. Russians also found that garlic has antibiotic properties—they commonly refer to garlic as "Russian penicillin." Russian clinics and hospitals use garlic extensively, mostly in the form of volatile extracts that are vaporized and inhaled.

During my travels in Russia, studying their health system and the native diets and their effects on health and longevity, I observed that Russian doctors, through the available channels of public health education, advise people to eat lots of garlic and onions as a health-promoting and disease-preventing measure. It is not uncommon to see Russians munching on a large onion the way we eat apples. And, the fact that they eat lots of garlic can be evidenced by the unmistakable aroma every time you mingle with the crowds.

Russian scientists studied the antibiotic effect of garlic or garlic extracts on infected wounds of 30 rabbits. After treatment of the wounds with phytocides of garlic and the other plant hormones, they noticed an increase of RNA and DNA levels in the experimental animals as well as noticeable inhibition in bacterial growth and speeded healing of wounds.[17]

ANTIBACTERIAL AND ANTIFUNGAL PROPERTIES OF GARLIC

Numerous studies demonstrate that garlic juice exhibits strong antibacterial and antifungal properties. Due to those properties, garlic has been widely known as a blood purifier.

Nobel Prize Laureate, Dr. Arthur Stoll, established in the 1940's the antibiotic and bactericidal effects of garlic and ascribed this power to the alliin, a sulfur-containing amino acid present in garlic.[8]

In Russian studies by Drs. D. B. Dubova [18] and E. P. Leskinov,[19] it was established that a number of fungus diseases responded to treatment with garlic juice. According to Indian studies by Datta and others, the active factors in garlic, *allistatin I* and *allistatin II,* were found to be powerful agents against *Staphylococcus* and *Escherichia coli* (E. coli). Russian studies demonstrated that garlic extract was useful in the treatment of such disorders as chronic colitis, gastritis, grippe, and whooping cough.

ANTICANCER PROPERTIES OF GARLIC

Garlic preparations of various kinds, mostly in natural form, but also as extracts or juices, have been used successfully against cancer, both in animal and human studies.

In animal studies by Weisberger and Pensky of Western Reserve University, as reported in *Science,* 1957,[20] mice injected with cancer cells died within 16 days. When cancer cells were treated with garlic extract and injected into the animals, no deaths occurred for a period of 6 months. In other studies, feeding fresh garlic to female mice completely inhibited the development of mammary tumors.[21]

And, in Russian studies, garlic preparation was found not only to retard tumor growth in animals, but also in humans.[22]

Germanium and Cancer

At a recent Cancer Control Convention in Los Angeles, Dr. K. Asai, of Japan, reported on his extensive studies of the trace mineral, germanium, which has been found to have both preventive and curative effects on cancer.[23] Garlic is one of the best natural sources of germanium. Although there are many active factors in garlic that have been shown to possess therapeutic effects, the germanium, according to Japanese research, may be one of the most important factors as far as cancer is concerned. The reason for making such an assertion is based on empirical evidence of the low cancer incidence among peoples like Chinese and Koreans, who eat large amounts of garlic daily. Also, the results of animal experiments conducted at the Tokyo Medical University Laboratory of Hygienics show that garlic in the daily diet can help prevent formation of cancer. Injection of cancer cells were given to two groups of rats. One group received garlic as an addition to the diet, while the control group received no garlic. Although cancer developed in the group that received no garlic, the garlic-fed group remained totally free from cancer.

GARLIC: THE MIRACLE HEALER

In the controlled and reliable clinical studies—animal as well as human—mentioned above and reported in major medical journals world-wide in the last couple of decades, garlic has been shown to have almost miraculous preventive and/or therapeutic properties in the treatment of a variety of diseases. Here is a partial list of ailments that have been successfully treated by raw garlic or garlic extracts:

high blood pressure
atherosclerosis
tuberculosis
diabetes
arthritis
cancer
hypoglycemia

bronchitis
asthma (garlic juice mixed with comfrey juice)
whooping cough
pneumonia
common cold
allergies
intestinal worms
intestinal putrefaction and gas
parasitic diarrhea
dysentery
insomnia

In the treatment of the above-mentioned diseases, garlic has been used by biologically oriented physicians singularly or as an effective adjunct to other nutritional and biological modalities.

Personally, I have used garlic very successfully in my clinical practice to treat patients with metabolic diarrhea, parasitic diarrhea, intestinal putrefaction, intestinal worms, dysentery, dyspepsia, asthma, and high blood pressure. I have found that one of the most effective ways to arrest an approaching sore-throat-type of cold is to cut a large clove of garlic in half and keep both halves in the mouth for several hours, if possible.

OTHER CLINICAL USES OF GARLIC

In addition to the long list of diseases mentioned above, in which garlic treatment has resulted in clinically observable success, there are many other health disorders that have been reported to be favorably affected by garlic treatment:

Eye burns. An emulsion of naphthalene ointment with phytocides of garlic and onions showed a high effectiveness in treatment of eye burns.[24]

Lip and mouth diseases. Russian doctors, Sergejev and Leonov, have reported treatment of 194 cases of lip and mouth disorders. They placed garlic paste on a gauze and applied to the affected area, securing it in place with tape for 8–12 hours. Complete healing was observed in over 90 percent of the cases in such disorders as leukoplakia (white spots), hyperkeratosis (a horny swelling) and fissures and ulcers of the lip.[25]

Coagulation disorders. It has been demonstrated in clinical studies by coagulographic technique that garlic contains blood anticoagulant constituents.[26]

Upset stomach. Garlic contains an active component called gastroenteric allichalon which has a sedative action, due to its delaying effect upon excessive motor activity of the stomach and of the intestines.[27]

Hyperemia
Grippe
Sciatica
Chronic Colitis
Gastritis
Whooping Cough. All the above conditions were successfully treated with garlic by Russian doctors and the results reported in Russian medical literature. In most cases, the doctor's conclusion was that garlic extract and other preparations were more effective than penicillin, or compared favorably with sulfa therapy.[28]

Beriberi. The daily use of garlic oil (10 mg.) prevented beriberi even when thiamine-deficient diets were fed. Also, garlic administration produced recovery from diagnosed beriberi.[29]Garlic contains a biologically active thiamine, *allithiamine.* Thiamine (vitamin B_1) deficiency is a major cause of beriberi.

Pimples. It has been reported by many laymen and doctors that pimples disappear without scars when rubbed several times a day with raw garlic. The blood of the person, however, must also be purified; therefore, garlic should be also taken internally in order for the pimples to remain cleared up.[30]

Emphysema. Small amounts of garlic juice added to fresh vegetable juices has helped many patients with emphysema.

Athletes' foot. A variety of fungus infections, such as athletes' foot, responded to garlic treatment. Garlic should be taken internally, as well as applied directly to the affected parts as a dusting powder or oil.

Worms. Garlic has been used for this purpose since early history by Chinese, Greeks, Romans, Hindus, Babylonians, as well as by many modern biological practitioners. Both fresh garlic and garlic oil are effective. For those who do not like the taste of garlic and refuse to eat it (children, especially), an ancient method of garlic medication may be the answer: Place a couple cloves of fresh garlic in each shoe—yes, shoe! As the child walks, the garlic is crushed and the worm-killing garlic oil is absorbed by the skin and carried by the blood into the intestines. Garlic possesses a powerful penetrative force. Within 10 minutes of its being rubbed on the skin, its fragrance can be detected in the breath.[31]

Constipation. The regular eating of a moderate amount of garlic, especially mixed with onions and such leafy vegetables as kale, parsley, and comfrey, can help relieve even stubborn cases of chronic constipation. The allicin in garlic passes into the large intestine with other undigestible materials and there is decomposed by the action of bacteria. Allicin itself stimulates the peristaltic movement of the intestinal walls, and, thus, promotes better bowel action.[32] Some people with persistent, long-standing constipation, may need large doses of garlic to bring about relief. Occasionally, garlic may cause diarrhea. This is always temporary and is brought on by eating too much raw garlic. Note, however, that even persistent cases of chronic diarrhea, especially of the parasitic, bacterial kind, can be effectively treated with garlic.

Intestinal disorders. The *Medical Record,* June, 1941, carried a report by E. Weiss, M.D., of Chicago, who used garlic in treatment of 22 patients with a known history of intestinal disorders. Headaches, mild diarrhea, gas, and other symptoms of intestinal disorders disappeared during the garlic treatment. But the most important result of garlic administration was that the intestinal flora of the patients was completely changed. Intestinal flora are the bacteria living in the digestive tract. Some of these are beneficial and help in the digestion of food and synthesis of certain vitamins. Some are harmful bacteria which cause putrefaction in the intestines and contribute to autotoxemia and the resultant ill health. As a result of garlic treatment, the beneficial bacteria were increased in all the patients, while the harmful, disease-causing bacteria, decreased. Many other studies confirm that garlic combats intestinal toxemia and improves digestion and assimilation of food.

Colds. Garlic has been used for centuries as an effective preventive as well as curative treatment for colds. Medical science considered this as superstition and "old wives' tales" of ignorant peasants. Finally, the effectiveness of garlic as a cold remedy was scientifically tested by Dr. J. Klosa, M.D., and reported in *Medical Monthly* in March, 1950. The report said that all kinds of cold symptoms—grippe, sore throats, runny nose, fever, cough, rhinitis, etc.—were cut short in every case. All patients showed a distinct lessening of the period of the disease as well as of convalescence required. Both raw garlic and garlic preparations are effective.

Well, isn't this an impressive list of health conditions and disorders that can be corrected or relieved by the lowly, odoriferous little bulb of garlic! Perhaps the old folk tale wasn't far off that declared:

> "Eat onions in March and garlic in May—
> Then the rest of the year, your doctor can play."

PESTICIDAL PROPERTIES OF GARLIC

Two entomologists from the University of California, Drs. Elden L. Reeves, and Shankar V. Amonkar proved by their studies that garlic is an effective pesticide.[33,34] Using what they refer to as a "crude extract of garlic," they discovered that it caused 100% mortality in five species of mosquito larvae when used in such small doses as 200 p.p.m. (parts per million).

The California researchers used a crude methanolic extract of commercially available dehydrated garlic, called instant minced garlic, and also a more refined form obtained from freshly reconstituted dehydrated garlic by steam distillation. Both of these materials were used against larvae of a number of mosquitoes, including *Culex peus, Aedes*, and even against a field-collected larvae of highly insecticide-resistant strains of *A. nigromaculis* from Tulare and Kern counties in California. A 100% mortality rate was obtained against all larvae with the crude garlic extract at the concentration of 200 p.p.m. or above, and 90% mortality if concentration was 100 p.p.m. The steam distilled garlic oil fraction gave even better results: 100% mortality at 20 p.p.m. for laboratory-bred larvae and 30 p.p.m. for field-collected, highly insecticide-resistant larvae. They found that the oil fraction is $12\frac{1}{2}$ times as effective as crude garlic extract.[34]

Isn't it ironic that we have been told all these years that it would be fatal to outlaw DDT because we have to have it to kill mosquitoes! But, I guess it is easier to produce a chemical concoction than to grow garlic on a mass scale. The fact that DDT also kills people doesn't seem to enter the chemical boys' minds.

By the way, organic gardeners around the world have known for years that planting rows of garlic plants between rows

27

of vegetables or flowers which are specifically vulnerable to insect attacks, such as roses, tomatoes, potatoes, cabbage, etc., will prevent insect infestation and protect the plants. One of my friends soaks raw mashed garlic in large vats of water, then sprinkles it on the plants—with excellent results of total protection!

ANIMAL DISEASES AND GARLIC

Volatile fractions of aqueous and alcholic extracts of garlic were used effectively to treat animals infested with ticks, which are the carriers of a deadly disease, encephalitis. The ticks stopped increasing in about 20 minutes and dried after about 30 minutes.[35] Garlic showed a striking repellent effect against new infestations.

Hoof and mouth disease in cattle was also treated successfully with garlic.[36]

ANTIOXIDANT PROPERTY OF GARLIC

Like onions, marjoram, and green chilies, garlic is known to possess an antioxidant property, and is used for this purpose in food preparation in many countries, as for example, in the preparation of ghee. Ghee is a heated butter that is very stable in terms of rancidity. An Indian study showed that garlic exhibited a high antioxidant property as determined by the peroxide values of the products by the swift stability test.[41] Garlic restrained the development of all characteristic indexes of rancidity (acidity, peroxides, iodine No., etc.). Garlic retained its antioxidant property for a half year after harvesting.

GARLIC: POWERFUL DETOXIFIER

Perhaps the most clearly observable effect of garlic in the treatment of most diseases is its detoxifying effect on the body. Whether due to the factors mentioned above, or some other unidentified factors, garlic is a powerful detoxifier. It neutralizes toxins present in the digestive tract and eliminative organs, as well as in the blood, and has a beneficial effect on the function of the liver, kidneys, nervous system, and circulatory system. Garlic, being an anti-toxin, also strengthens the body's defenses against allergens, and is, therefore, used in the treatment of allergies, asthma, and hypoglycemia.[15,16]

An excellent study that demonstrates the protective, detoxifying effect of garlic was made in Japan by H. Sumiyoshi, B.S., and S. Kitahara, Dr. Med. Sc. They fed one group of rats a purified diet plus 5% sodium cyclamate. The rats showed growth retardation, lack of weight gain, poor grooming, extensive diarrhea, and varying degrees of alopecia (hair loss). The second group of rats was fed the same purified diet, and the same 5% sodium cyclamate, but it was also given 10% special garlic preparation. The garlic preparation with its detoxifying property apparently counteracted the toxic effects of sodium cyclamate, and the rats grew healthy and strong to almost twice the size of the rats that did not receive garlic.

Our food, air, water, and environment are heavily contaminated with various poisons and toxic, man-made chemicals, such as food additives and preservatives, artificial colorings and flavorings, artificial sweeteners (such as cyclamate), chemical fertilizers, pesticides, etc. It is good to know that the regular use of garlic, or garlic preparations, can help to neutralize these toxins and protect our bodies from their harmful effects.

HEAVY METAL POISONING AND GARLIC

The threat to our health from environmental poisons, and specifically heavy metals, is increasing every day. Lead, mercury, cadmium, arsenic, and copper poisoning are becoming epidemic. Lead and mercury come mostly from polluted air plus industrial and medical uses, such as lead-containing paint and mercury-containing amalgam dental fillings. Contaminated fish are also a common source of mercury poisoning. Copper enters our bodies usually from copper water pipes, commonly used in plumbing.

Heavy metal poisoning is difficult to treat. Chelation treatment is the only known medical treatment that is effective in detoxifying the body of heavy metals. Now, the Japanese study conducted by Drs. Ikezoe and Kitahara, shows that Kyolic, a raw garlic extract developed in Japan, is effective in protecting the body from the toxic effects of the heavy metal poisoning.[39]

Dr. Kitahara and his co-workers, Ikezoe and Yamada, conducted controlled studies on animals (rabbits) and humans. The method of study was: observation of release of potassium and hemoglobin by heavy metals from erythrocytes, and destruction of erythrocyte membrane. The conclusion of the study was that garlic preparation prevented the poisoning effect arising from heavy metals and protected the erythrocyte membrane from destruction.

In another study, conducted in Russia, a drug made from garlic extract was given to workers in industrial plants who were suffering from chronic lead poisoning. The daily doses of garlic improved the symptoms of chronic lead poisoning and lowered the high porphyrin levels in the urine. The preparation also normalized the elevated blood pressure in the majority of workers.[40] Russian researchers believe that the efficacy of the garlic preparation is due to garlic's high content of sulfur compounds.

The following charts show the effectiveness of garlic in binding with heavy metals in the system and helping to eliminate them from the body.

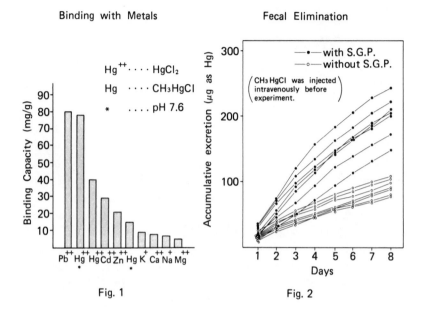

Fig. 1   Fig. 2

Fig. 1 on the left shows the binding capacity of garlic preparation with such heavy metals as lead (Pb), organic and inorganic mercury (Hg), and Cadmium (Cd). Note that garlic seems to have a selective attraction to dangerous metals such as lead, mercury, and cadmium, sparing the needed and beneficial minerals such as calcium, magnesium, potassium, and zinc.

Fig. 2 on the right shows that rats injected with mercury intravenously before the experiment, eliminated it with feces 2–3 times faster than the control group.

The garlic preparation used in the experiment (SGP) was the Japanese garlic extract, Leopin (known as Kyolic in the United States). The study was conducted by Dr. S. Kitahara, H. Sumiyoshi, and K. Kamiota.

These studies may have a far-reaching effect, as it is becoming more and more difficult to avoid deadly toxic metals, especially lead and mercury, in our poisoned environment.

HOW AND WHY GARLIC WORKS

Although there is plenty of empirical and clinical evidence that garlic is effective both in prevention as well as treatment of disease, scientific studies are meager as to what specific factors in garlic are responsible for these beneficial effects. At present, it is generally considered by most researchers that the sulfur-containing compounds in garlic, especially allicin, aliin, cycroalliin, and diallyldisulphide—there are 33 such compounds isolated as of now—are the most active substances. I am sure that future studies will reveal more "unidentified factors" in garlic in addition to the factors which are presently known. For example, the famous Finnish Nobel Prize winning scientist, Dr. A. I. Virtanen, in his thorough biochemical analysis of onions, discovered 14 new beneficial substances.

At present, research and clinical observations quoted previously have shown the following active factors being present in garlic (Allium Sativum):

- **Allicin,** the substance in garlic that is believed to be largely responsible for garlic's antibacterial and anti-inflammatory effects. Allicin is also the odorous factor in the garlic.

- **Alliin,** a sulfur-containing amino acid in garlic from which allicin is made by the action of the enzyme alliinase. Russian studies ascribed the antibiotic effect of garlic to its alliin content.

- **Diallyldisulphide-oxide,** a chemical compound into which allicin is changed in the system. The essential oil of garlic contains 6% allylpropyldisulphide and 60% diallyldisulphide. The cholesterol- and lipid-lowering effect of garlic is attributed to the presence of this factor.[9,37]

- **Gurwitch rays,** the mitogenetic radiation factor that stimulates cell growth and has a rejuvenating stimulating effect on all body functions.[2]

- **Anti-hemolytic factor,** responsible for its beneficial effect in the treatment of anemia. Note: this factor was proven to be present only in allicin-free garlic preparations, such as Kyolic or Leopin.[11]

- **Anti-arthritic factor,** as shown in Japanese studies at Fukuyama Hospital.[12]

- **Sugar-regulating factor,** which makes garlic useful as an adjunct in the treatment of both diabetes and hypoglycemia.[14]

- **Antioxidant factor.** Garlic was shown to inhibit peroxidation (rancidity) of foods, and thus, can be used as a natural preservative.[41]

- **Anti-coagulant factor.** According to clinical studies, garlic contains effective blood anti-coagulant factors.[26]

- **Allithiamine.** Garlic is an excellent source of biologically active compounds of vitamin B_1. Japanese researchers (Matsukawa et al.)[38] have isolated from garlic a substance, allithiamine, which is formed by the action of vitamin B_1 on alliin. This component has been found to have beneficial therapeutic properties and to be effective, among other things, in preventing and curing beriberi.

- **Selenium.** Garlic is also an excellent source of biologically active selenium, and it is believed that garlic's anti-atherosclerotic property (preventing platelet adhesion and clot formation) is due to its high selenium content.[8] Selenium also normalizes blood pressure and has been shown to protect against infections.

THE CHEMICAL AND NUTRITIONAL COMPOSITION OF GARLIC

As I have mentioned before, the healing effect of garlic has been attributed to various specific factors present in the garlic bulb, such as allicin and alliin, which are among 33 other sulfur-containing compounds, plus the ultra-violet radiation—the Gurwitch rays. Garlic is rich in sulfur-containing amino acids, 1-cystein and methionine. As soon as garlic is crushed or eaten, the alliin ($CH-CH_2-\overset{\displaystyle O}{\underset{\displaystyle}{S}}-CH_2\overset{\displaystyle NH_2}{\underset{\displaystyle}{C}}H-COOH$) is converted to allicin ($C_3H_5-\overset{\displaystyle}{\underset{\displaystyle O}{S}}-S-C_3H_5$) by the action of the enzyme alliinase. The essential oil of garlic contains 60% allicin. Allicin is the strong, odorous substance of the garlic. But it does not develop until the garlic bulb is crushed and the enzyme is released. The reason that *cooked* garlic does not have a strong odor is because the enzyme alliinase is destroyed in cooking and, thus, the allicin is not developed. Since the allicin, or rather the diallyldisulphide ($C_3H_5-S-S-C_3H_5$) into which allicin is changed in the system (or in some special garlic preparations such as Kyolic), is only present in the raw state, it is important that garlic is used mostly in raw form, especially if therapeutic, not just culinary, effects are desired.

Many doctors, including David Stain, M.D., and E. Kotin, M.D.[42] who use garlic in their practice, suggested that because of the high therapeutic value, garlic must contain large amounts of vitamins, especially A, B, and C. However, my studies could not confirm this. Considering how small a quantity of garlic is normally consumed, as compared with other vegetables, garlic is a poor dietary source of vitamins A and C, but does contain a special kind of B_1 vitamin, allithiamine, which some researchers (Dr. Kitahara) consider to be of exceptional biological value. The leaves of garlic contain, however, large amounts of vitamins C and A.

The mineral content of garlic, on the other hand, is considerable. Garlic contains maganese, copper, iron, zinc, sulfur, calcium, aluminum, chlorine, germanium, and selenium. The sulfur content of garlic is one of the highest of all vegetables. The selenium content is most remarkable—in fact, garlic is the best-known natural source of selenium. On a wet basis, garlic contains 9.3 y/100 g. of selenium, which is 0.44 p.p.m. on a dry weight basis. Selenium is becoming more and more recognized as one of the most important trace elements in human nutrition. Garlic's antioxidant activity is probably due to its selenium content, since selenium is a strong antioxidant; its biological activity is closely related to vitamin E. Selenium may slow down aging processes by an inhibiting action on the formation of free radicals. This may explain why most of the centenarians whom I studied in Bulgaria and Russia are heavy garlic consumers. Selenium also can protect from toxic damage caused by mercury poisoning. As you can see, many of the best-known properties of garlic, such as antioxidant, anti-aging, and anti-toxin activity, may simply be due to its rich content of the miracle-working mineral, selenium. Brewer's yeast is another good source of selenium.

DELICIOUS GOURMET FOOD

In addition to having such miraculous preventive, protective, nutritional, and healing properties, garlic is also a most delicious food, enjoyed and treasured by most peoples around the world. Used wisely and in moderation, it can improve the nutritional quality as well as enhance the taste of many cooked dishes as well as raw salads. In French, Spanish, Italian, and Mexican cuisine, garlic is used in almost everything. One favorite Mexican dish is garlic soup—something like French onion soup, but made from garlic.

Personally, I use garlic in and on anything except fruit. My favorite dish is a raw vegetable salad with lots of tomatoes, avocados, and 2–3 finely chopped cloves of garlic. I also love garlic and cheese sandwiches. On a slice of dark sourdough rye bread, spread a layer of chopped raw garlic and cover with a thick slice of natural cheese of your choice. Delicious! And, of course, no soup is complete without some garlic or garlic powder.

GARLIC AND COMMON SENSE

So, to answer the question raised by the reader in the beginning of this book—is garlic a poison or a miracle food—don't let anyone confuse you! Garlic is most certainly a terrific health food as well as a miraculous medicine. In fact, as I said in the Introduction, garlic fulfills, more than any other food I know, Hippocrates' requirement of a perfect food—that our food should be our medicine—and our medicine should be our food.

But aside from all the scientific evidence presented in this book, perhaps the most effective, common-sense proof of garlic's harmlessness is the fact that Italians, Koreans, Russians, and Mexicans have been, and are now, using so much garlic in their daily diets, that if the scoffers and critics of garlic were right in their claims that garlic is poisonous, the traditional garlic eaters would all be sick or dead by now. Yet, they are some of the healthiest peoples on this planet! As far as the Italians are concerned, garlic and olive oil apparently can even counteract the negative effect of too much pasta!

"If he kissed you once, will he kiss you again?"

Now, I hear my readers complaining in unison: "Okay, okay! I believe you! I am convinced by the evidence you have presented, and it all makes sense to me. *But!* I am a social creature, I am married, I have a family, I work, I mingle with people. If I eat garlic the way you recommend, my marriage will be ruined, I will lose my job, and will never be able to come within six feet of anyone! It may be okay in Italy or Korea, but here, in the land of mouthwashes and deodorants, you just don't go around reeking of garlic."

It is true that in our culture, eating garlic may have social repercussions and impose some social limitations. Of course, there would be no problem if *everyone* ate garlic—like everyone in Italy does. Those who eat garlic themselves cannot detect the odor of garlic from others. It's just like smoking—those who smoke don't notice the objectionable odor of tobacco coming from others.

Usually, garlic, when used in cooking, does not leave garlic breath—only *raw* garlic does. Throughout the years, there have been several garlic and onion breath deodorizers, but none of them have proved to be 100% effective. Eating parsley or other chlorophyll-rich vegetables helps, but it does not remove the odor completely. Odorless garlic pills or garlic oil capsules? They are almost safe as far as breath is concerned, but even they do not pass the close-up test, such as kissing.

Great News From Japan!

Recently, I made an extensive tour of Japan where I studied their eating and living habits as well as presented several public and professional lectures on behalf of the International Academy of Biological Medicine. I learned many health secrets from the health-oriented Japanese, such as buckwheat soba, soy miso, and their many ways of eating large amounts of seaweed daily. But one of the most exciting items of health news I brought from Japan was actually not a part of their traditional diet at all—it was the new, completely odorless garlic preparation developed by the highly enterprising and ingenious Japanese. They have developed a garlic supplement called Kyolic (Kyo-Leopin in Japan, or Leopin in Canada) which retains all the traditional well-known medicinal and nutritional properties of raw garlic, *without garlic's odor.* By a special process, which involves curing garlic in huge vats for 20 months, without the use of heat, organically grown garlic loses its odor through a natural fermentation process. It is sold in liquid or tablet form and it has been available in Japan for some time, as one of the most widely used supplements. It has been tested for its therapeutic value by several research clinics in Japan and Australia, and it is approved by the Japanese equivalent of our FDA for preventive and therapeutic use. Best of all, Kyolic is now available in the United States and is sold in most health food stores. It is the only garlic product I know of that leaves absolutely no breath or body odor, even when taken in large doses.

Consequently, if on the basis of all the evidence presented in this book so far, you are convinced that garlic has a great health-improving, disease-preventing potential, and would like to incorporate it into your daily diet, but are afraid to do so because of possible social repercussions, you can safely enjoy garlic's traditional benefits by using Kyolic regularly. Or, train your whole family to eat garlic in its many natural forms every day, and associate yourself socially with other garlic eaters.

A suggestion: let's make garlic eating the new "in" thing (just like non-smoking or jogging) so that those of us who eat garlic regularly will not have to excuse ourselves for its delightful health-giving aroma.

QUESTIONS AND ANSWERS

Here are some other common questions I receive regarding garlic, which are not previously answered in this book:

How Much Garlic?

Q. How much raw garlic can one take each day? If I use garlic pills—how many should I take?

A. Only because you know that garlic is good for you doesn't mean that you can gorge on it in unlimited quantities. Remember, garlic is not so much a food as a condiment or seasoning, and should be used judiciously, the way other strong spices such as peppers, chilies, etc., are used. The excess of volatile oils in garlic may cause some unpleasant symptoms if used in extreme excess. Two or three small cloves of garlic in one meal are sufficient, possibly only one clove in most cases.

The garlic pills and other preparations should be taken as recommended in the directions on the label. Kyolic is usually taken in doses of 3–4 capsules twice a day; garlic oil pills usually 2–3 pills three times a day. The only exception to this limitation rule is when garlic is used in cooked form. When used in cooking, I don't know of any danger of consuming even large amounts, like several whole bulbs in garlic soup. When used as seasoning for salads, garlic should be used sparingly, as its flavor tends to overpower other more delicate scents and flavors of milder vegetables.

When To Take

Q. Can you tell me when I should take raw garlic, and also when to take pills or capsules: before meals, with meals, after meals, or between meals?

A. Raw garlic is best eaten with a vegetable meal, which in the Airola Optimum Diet is the evening meal. One or two cloves of garlic, finely chopped, added to a big, raw mixed vegetable salad, is one of the most delicious ways to eat garlic. As I said earlier, finely chopped garlic, spread on a slice of black rye bread and covered with butter and a slice of strong, natural cheese, such as aged cheddar, is another delightful way. Of course, any of the raw or cooked vegetables dishes can be spiked with garlic or garlic powder.

The capsules or pills are best taken *with meals;* whether right before, with, or right after the meal makes no difference. But, not between meals. If you take garlic pills or capsules only once a day, the evening (vegetable) meal is the best time. If garlic capsules are taken for therapeutic uses, in addition to taking them with meals, they can be taken at night before retiring.

Garlic Juice

Q. I drink a lot of vegetable juices every day. Could garlic be juiced together with the other vegetable juices and taken in that form?

A. Yes, this is one of the most effective ways to use garlic for therapeutic purposes. You can use a special garlic press (available at any department store) and squeeze a few drops of fresh garlic juice (from 1 or 2 cloves) directly into the freshly made vegetable juice: carrot, celery, beet, greens, etc. If used for asthma or emphysema, freshly made comfrey juice mixed with garlic juice is an excellent remedy. Remember, do not use too much—a few drops of garlic juice is all that is needed.

Where To Buy

Q. Garlic is something that I've never tasted in my life. Where do you buy fresh garlic and/or garlic supplements?

A. Fresh garlic (dried garlic bulbs) are sold in most supermarkets and in many health food stores. Garlic supplements, such as Kyolic or garlic oil pills, are sold in most health food stores.

Garlic Leaves

Q. I have had garlic planted in my garden for years, and have enjoyed it in my cooking. I've always wondered if the garlic leaves, like onion leaves, can be used for food, or are they toxic?

A. No, garlic leaves are not toxic; they are very edible and should not be wasted. When the garlic plant grows to about 8–10 inches high and develops as many as 8–10 leaves, the outside leaves (one at a time from each plant) can be picked and used in salads or in cooking. They are delicious and much milder in taste than the cloves of the bulb. They also contain a large amount of vitamins A and C.

How To Plant

Q. I would like to plant garlic in my garden next spring. How should I go about it?

A. Buy garlic bulbs from your grocer or health food store. Make sure the garlic cloves are hard and solid, not dried out. Separate the cloves from the bulb and plant each clove separately about ½ to 1 inch deep, 6 inches apart, in rows 6–8 inches apart. Just press clove, *with root end down,* into the ground and press the soil tightly around it, leaving it just barely visible.

Water every day for the first couple of weeks. Garlic grows well in practically any soil, and in any climate, from far north to the tropics. In the fall, when the leaves dry up and drop to the ground, pull the bulb out and dry outside in the shade for a few days until the roots are completely dry. After that, store inside in a dry place in a brown paper bag (not in a plastic bag). Do not store in the refrigerator. Garlic keeps best at room temperature. Under proper food storage conditions (dark and dry) garlic can be kept for a year. However, garlic's medicinal properties are most potent when it is fresh, and diminish drastically if the garlic is over 6 months old.

Garlic Soup

Q. I've heard about garlic soup. How do you make it?

A. Garlic soup is eaten in many countries. My experience with garlic soup is mostly from Mexico. I don't know exactly how Mexican chefs prepare it, but here is my own recipe for garlic soup—and it is delicious!

> Take one whole yellow or white onion and one whole garlic bulb. Wash and remove skins. Cut garlic cloves in half horizontally and chop onion into approximately ½ inch pieces. Place in a pot with 5 cups of water. Bring to a boil and simmer for 10 minutes. With a potato masher, mash the contents right in the pan, or place the contents in a blender and blend for 10 seconds, then place the contents back in the pan. Add 1 tsp. of vegetable broth powder and spices to taste. I use red chili (cayenne) and sea salt. Bring to a boil again. Add 2 raw eggs and beat rapidly with a wire whisk, so eggs will be well mixed. Serve at once. Makes 3–4 servings.

CONCLUSION

The empirical and scientific evidence presented in this publication shows that garlic is, indeed, a tremendously nutritious health food and a miraculous healing plant. It can truthfully be called "the king of the vegetable kingdom." Garlic, in its natural form, or in the form of special garlic pills, tablets, and other supplements should be incorporated in the Optimum Diet as one of the most beneficial and delicious natural seasonings and flavor enhancers. Garlic not only will improve and enrich the diet, but will help to improve your health, prevent disease, and prolong life.

REFERENCES

1. Adams, Ruth, and Murray, Frank, *Health Foods,* Larchmont Books, New York, 1975.
2. Airola, Paavo, *Are You Confused?,* Health Plus Publishers, Phoenix, Arizona, 1971.
3. Coon, Nelson, *Using Plants For Healing,* Heartside Press.
4. Piotrowski, F. G., *Praxis,* July 1, 1948.
5. "Nutrition News Byline," *Alive,* Canadian Journal of Health and Nutrition, 12, 1977.
6. Debray and Loeper, *Bull. Soc. Med.,* 37, 1032, 1921.
7. Petkov, V., Deut. Apotheker-Z., 106 (51), 1861, 1966.
8. Passwater, Richard, *Supernutrition for Healthy Hearts,* the Dial Press, New York, N.Y., 1977.
9. Augusti, K. T., and Mathew, P. T., *Indian Journal of Exp. Biology,* 1973. Also, *Experientia,* 30,5, 1974.
10. *Experientia,* 15, 5, 1974, p. 469.
11. Halwax, K., Research paper published by Wakunaga Pharmaceutical Co., Hiroshima, Japan.
12. Wakunaga Pharmaceutical Company, report to the author, with detailed study data.
13. Prasan, D. N., et al., *Indian Journal of Med. Res.,* 54 (6), 582, 1966.
14. Jain, R. C., et al., *Lancet,* Dec. 29, 1973.
15. Airola, Paavo, *Hypoglycemia: A Better Approach,* Health Plus Publishers, Phoenix, Arizona, 1977.
16. Brahmachari, H. D., and Augusti, K. T., *Journal of Pharmacology,* 14, 254, 1962.
17. Tagiev, G. A., *Azerb. Med. Zh.* 44 (4), 82, 1967.
18. Dubova, D. B., *Mikrobiologiya,* 19, 222, 1950.
19. Leskinov, E. P., *Byull. Eksperim. Biologiskoy Mediciny,* 21 (1) 70, 1947.
20. Weisberger, A. S., and Pensky, J., *Science,* 126, 1112, Nov. 29, 1957.
21. Kroening, K., *Acta Unio. Intern. Contra Cancium,* 20, 855, 1964.
22. Romanyuk, N. M., *Ukrainskaya Biokhim. Zh.,* 24, 53, 1952.
23. Asai, K., report at Cancer Control Convention, Los Angeles, California, July 3, 1977. The tape of Dr. Asai's report can be obtained from Cancer Control Society, 2043 N. Berendo, Los Angeles, California 90027.
24. Safarli, S. R., *Vestn. Oftalmol.,* 34 (6), 17, 1955.

25. Sergejev, D. M., and Leonov, I. D., *The Encyclopedia for Healthful Living,* Rodale Press, Pennsylvania, 1960.
26. Lorenzovelazquez, B., et al., *Arch. Inst. Farmocolog. Exp.* 8, 28, 1956.
27. Damrau, F., and Ferguson, E. A., *Rev. Gastroenterol.,* 16, 411, 1949.
28. Ikram, M., *Pakistan J. Sci. Ind. Res.,* vol. 15, No. 1–2, February-April, 1972.
29. Zentat, Susatoh, *Vitamins,* 5,306, 1952.
30. Several personal communications to the author.
31. Airola, Paavo, *How to Get Well,* Health Plus Publishers, Phoenix, Arizona, 1974.
32. *Garlic Therapy,* "Specific effects," p. 45.
33. *Chemical and Engineering News,* February 16, 1970.
34. Amonkar, S. V., and Reeves, E. L., *Journal of Econ. Entomol.,* 63, 1172, 1972.
35. Catar, G., *Bratislav. Lekarske Listy,* 34, 1004, 1954.
36. Schiefer, H., *Austrian Patent,* 176,065, Sept. 10, 1953.
37. Parry, E. J., *Chemistry of Essential Oils and Artificial Perfumes,* Scott, Greenwood and Son, London, 1922, vol. 1., p. 92.
38. Matzukawa, et al., *Journal of Pharmaceutical Society of Japan,* 72, 1585, 1952.
39. Ikezoe, T., and Kitahara, S., Medical Journal, *Kiso-to-Rinsho,* Japan, March, 1975.
40. Petrov, V., et al., *Gigiena Truda i Prof. Zabolevaniya,* 9 (4), 42, 1955.
41. Dhar, D. C., *Journal of Indian Chemical Society,* Ind. & News Ed. 14, 175, 1951.
42. Article in *New York Physician,* Sept. 1937.

WHAT CRITICS, DOCTORS AND READERS SAY ABOUT

PAAVO AIROLA'S BOOKS

Dr. S. Marshall Fram, M.D., Long Beach, Ca.: "Your book, "How To Get Well", is tremendous and extremely helpful; I keep it on my desk and refer to it constantly."

Linda Clark, M.A., Author, Carmel, Ca.: "How To Get Well" is extremely practical and helpful for the reader, and a giant example of research and work. I will refer to it many times, giving you credit all the way.... Many thanks, and congratulations."

Dr. L. E. Essén,, M.D., Sweden: "I am congratulating you for your pioneer work. Your work will contribute to the freedom of thought and of therapeutic alternatives—and, thus, to the improvement of the health standards in your country."

F. C. Winters, Phoenix: "I feel that your fasting book is a masterpiece. I have fasted many times in the past on water, but your juice fasting method is superior—I am on my 28th day of a juice fast, and feel great."

Dr. E. W. Conroy, New Zealand: "In all sincerity, I find that your books, particularly "Health Secrets From Europe" and "There *Is* A Cure For Arthritis", are my very best references on the many aspects of health, and they have been most helpful to me and my practice of any that I have gotten—and I have an extensive library. I find that "Are You Confused?" has straightened out a lot of questions in my.mind."

Dr. J. P. Hutchins, M.D., Wilmington, Ca.: "Dr. Airola's new book, "Hypoglycemia: A Better Approach", is an important contribution to the betterment of health, not only in this country, but around the world. It will revolutionize the treatment of hypoglycemia and will undoubtedly be used as a textbook in medical schools. In my opinion, Dr. Paavo Airola is the leading nutritionist in the world today—in the depth and scope of his knowledge."

Dr. Mary Ann Kibler, M.D., Corry, Pa.: "You deserve a great deal of credit for your very fine and informative books."

Betty Lee Morales, Nutrition Consultant, Los Angeles, Ca.: "How To Get Well" is wonderful.... This do-it-yourself sort of book is what the public is hungry for. No one deserves more than yourself the success you are having."

Ebba Waerland, Author-healer, Switzerland: "Thank you for your wonderful books. I am so happy to know that you are spreading the important message all over the world, which will show the suffering mankind the way to better health and happiness."

Scott S. Smith, Editor, "Vegetarian World", Los Angeles, Ca.: "Dr. Airola is America's foremost nutritionist and an acknowledged authority on holistic healing and biological medicine, who is in the unique position of having his ideas received favorably by a growing number of medical doctors."

Dr. H. Rudolph Alsleben, M.D., Anaheim, Ca.: "Your book, "How To Get Well", is sensational! I am impressed with the way you conceived and constructed it, with your fabulous and expert presentation of the philosophy of biological medicine and with common and academic sense that it makes.... You rendered a great service to a disease-ridden mankind."

Morris Halio, Lantana, Fl.: "I have read all of your books and regard you as the ultimate authority on health matters. "How To Get Well" is my nutrition Bible."

Robert Yaller, Author, Venice, Ca.: "We think your book, "Are You Confused?", is a masterpiece. It should be a *must* reading for everyone who wants to get a good idea on how to achieve real health."

Roy Garrison, Herbalist, Honolulu, Hi.: "We have just received "Hypoglycemia: A Better Approach." In our 54 years of study of health and healing, we can enthusiastically and honestly say that your book is, by far, the best book written on the subject."

Dr. M. O. Garten, Author, San Jose, Ca.: "I wish to compliment you on your brilliant and dynamic presentations of contemporary health problems and how they can be overcome in a most logical and convincing sequence. I have received great pleasure and stimulation from reading your books and feel you have given to the people of the Western world some priceless teachings which they are so pathetically in need of."

Dr. W. D. Currier, M.D., Pasadena, Ca.: "Your service to mankind cannot be overestimated. You are a leader in the natural health field and your books are invaluable both for laymen and professionals. Keep up the good work!"

Robert G. Wallace, St. Croix, V.I.: "Your book "How To Get Well" is the best health book in over the 100 health books that I have read.

Jon Bjornstad, Suitland, Md.: "Your book, "Are You Confused?", speaks straight and strong and true. I have been pursuing health for several years, but nothing I've read or heard had the ring of truth like your books. Following your advice I feel remarkable improvement in my health. Thank you, I praise you highly!"

Dr. Kathleen M. Power, D.C., Pasadena, Ca.: "Dr. Airola is not only the most knowledgeable, but also the most honest writer of them all."

Richard Barmakian, Nutritionist, Pasadena, Ca.: "How To Get Well" firmly establishes Dr. Airola as the most outstanding nutritionist in the world today."

Dr. Harvey Walker, M.D., Ph.D., Clayton, Mo.: "My patients and I thank you for publishing your findings, especially in the most useful book, "How To Get Well".

Dr. R. Huckabay, D.C., N.D., Los Angeles, Ca.: "Your book, "Are You Confused?", is the most important health book ever published."

Dr. William H. Khoe, M.D., Sun Valley, Ca.: "The best and most effective treatment for low blood sugar that I know of is outlined in Dr. Airola's book, "Hypoglycemia: A Better Approach". Up to eighty percent of my patients have low blood sugar and I treat them with the Airola Diet, with excellent results. The Airola Diet is far superior to the traditional high-protein diet."

Dr. David R. Anderson, M.A., N.D., Wheeling, Illinois "I have recently purchased your book, HOW TO GET WELL. I want to commend you for a very excellent book which will be a valuable guide in any physician's office."

Rev. Robert Strecker, Los Angeles, California "I stayed up all night reading your book . . . It's terrific."

Dr. C. Serritella, D.C., Caribou, Maine "I find your book, "Are You Confused?", excellent in every way . . . I believe the last chapter, Biological Medicine, is worth the price of the book alone."

Audry Smith, Reg. Therapist. Escondido, California "No doubt in my mind about it— you are the Number One nutritionist and the most knowledgeable health writer."

Dr. Louis Junker, Professor of Economics, Western Michigan University "Please send me a copy of Paavo Airola's HOW TO GET WELL. I am considering one or two of his books emphasizing biological medicine as text books in my Honors Class on nutrition-health relationship. I know of no better author on such matters."

(There are hundreds of similar unsolicited comments in publishers' files.)

ABOUT THE AUTHOR

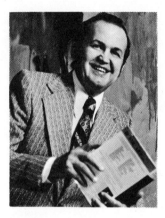

Paavo Airola, Ph.D., N.D., is an internationally recognized nutritionist, naturopathic physician, lecturer, and an award-winning author. He studied nutrition, biochemistry, and biological medicine in Europe and spent many years of research and study in European biological clinics and research centers. He is considered to be the leading authority on biological medicine and wholistic approach to healing in the United States. He lectures extensively, and worldwide, both to professionals and laymen, holding yearly educational seminars for physicians. He has recently lectured at the Stanford University Medical School.

Dr. Airola is the author of eleven widely-read books, notably his two international best-sellers, *Are You Confused?* and *How To Get Well.* The American Academy of Public Affairs issued Dr. Airola the Award of Merit for his book, *There Is A Cure For Arthritis. Are You Confused?* is heralded by many nutritionists, doctors, and critics as "the most important health book ever published," "a must reading for every sincere health seeker."

His comprehensive handbook on natural healing, *How To Get Well,* is the most authoritative and practical manual on biological medicine in print. It outlines complete nutritional, herbal, and other alternative biological therapies for all of our most common ailments and is used as a textbook in several universities and medical schools. It is regarded as a reliable reference manual by doctors, researchers, nutritionists, and students of health, nutrition, and biological medicine.

Dr. Airola's newest book, *Hypoglycemia: A Better Approach,* has revolutionized the concept of and the therapeutic approach to this insidious, complex, and devastating affliction which has assumed epidemic proportions.

Dr. Airola is President of the International Academy of Biological Medicine; a member of the International Naturopathic Association; and a member of the International Society for Research on Civilization Diseases and Environment, the prestigious forum for world-wide research, founded by Dr. Albert Schweitzer. He is listed in *The Directory of International Biography, The Blue Book, The Men of Achievement, Who's Who In American Art,* and *Who's Who in the West.*